Thyroid Health

Ultimate Guide that Will Cure Your Thyroid Problems

3rdEdition

Lucas Ether

Table Of Contents

information is without contract or any type of guarantee assurance.

The trademarks that are used are without any consent, and the publication of the trademark is without permission or backing by the trademark owner. All trademarks and brands within this book are for clarifying purposes only and are the owned by the owners themselves, not affiliated with this document.

Introduction

I want to thank you and congratulate you for downloading the book, "The Ultimate Guide to Heal Your Thyroid Third Edition!".

There are different types of thyroid problems and each one has a different cause and treatment. Thyroid problems can produce undesirable symptoms, including low energy, irritability and unintentional weight gain (or loss).

This book gives more information about other common types of thyroid disorder. The thyroid gland is an integral part of the body and it is also linked with other organs and systems as well. This book's second edition also discusses factors that can affect your thyroid health like those related to your gut, blood sugar and adrenal glands. This will help you understand the correlation between the thyroids and other systems in your body. Taking care of your overall health can increase your chances of recovery and make the healing process faster.

Fortunately, there are a lot of treatment options for people with thyroid problems. Conventional medicine and drugs are available to relieve symptoms, while some procedures like surgery and radioactive iodine can ultimately render the thyroid gland non-functional.

Some people can also opt for natural remedies, from using herbs to incorporating exercise to help keep their thyroid healthy. This book provides tips on what food to eat and what to avoid, depending on the type of thyroid problem.

Remember that different thyroid problems may require different treatments. Make sure to consult your doctor about any treatment option that you want to try. Anti-thyroid medication can also interact with other medications so be careful in adding any non-prescription drug into your treatment plan.

Maintaining a healthy lifestyle that incorporates nutrient-dense food and exercise can do a lot of good for your thyroid. Keeping your body generally healthy prevents further complications and hampers disease progression. Coping with stress can also help keep you emotionally and mentally stable. Use this book as a guide to make healthy choices, for the sake of keeping your thyroid in tiptop shape.

This book contains proven steps as well as strategies on how to cure your thyroid problems and maintain it for life.

Thanks again for downloading this book, I hope you enjoy it!

Chapter 1:
Thyroid Problems

The thyroid gland is an organ that is located at the neck. It is a butterfly-shaped gland that lies at the bottom of the Adam's apple and in front of the windpipe. It has two lobes that are connected by a bridge.

A normal size thyroid is small enough that it cannot be felt. The thyroid secretes hormones that help the body perform certain functions – such as balancing body temperature, influencing metabolism, and inhibiting growth and development. Thyroid development is especially important in the brain development of infants.

Identifying Thyroid Problems

Doctors test the hormone levels in the blood to determine if a person is suffering from a thyroid problem. The levels of thyroid-stimulating hormone in your body will indicate the cause of your thyroid problem.

Causes

There are many causes of thyroid problems, and here are some of them:

- Grave disease is an auto immune condition that can lead to excessive hormone production. It can also overwork the thyroid gland.

- Toxic adenomas manifest when nodules develop inside the thyroid gland, causing it to secrete too much hormones. This disrupts the chemical balance in the body – sometimes even causing goiters to form.

- Inflammations in the thyroid can make excess hormones leak outwards. This can cause temporary hyperthyroidism.

- Malfunctions in the pituitary gland may also cause thyroid gland problems.

- Overexposure to lithium can cause hypothyroidism.

- When part of the thyroid gland is removed because of hyperthyroidism, it becomes susceptible to hypothyroidism.

Symptoms of Thyroid Problems

Millions of people suffer from thyroid problems. There are certain symptoms that serve as telltale signs of a developing thyroid problem, such as:

- Muscle or joint pain, which is usually felt around the joints and muscles. Carpal tunnel syndrome can also develop in the arms and hands.

- Excessive hair loss

- A part of the throat (or the entire neck) swells and enlarges. This is also a sign of goiter, which can be linked to thyroid problems.

- Dry, thick, and scaly skin is among the symptoms of hypothyroidism. People suffering from hyperthyroidism have thin and fragile skin.

- Bowel problems

- Infertility is sometimes associated with thyroid problems

Treatment for Thyroid Problems

For thyroid disorders that lead to hormone production concerns, both medical and holistic methods are effective in restoring the natural balance of hormones. Most conventional treatments make use of medication. Make sure that you undergo a medical for the sake of knowing whether you really have a thyroid disorder.

Chapter 2:
Thyroid Problem Treatments

It is best to consult your doctor before administering any type of treatment. A doctor can make a proper diagnosis, and come up with a treatment plan that suits you perfectly.

Treatments for Hyperthyroidism

Hyperthyroidism is a condition where the thyroid produces too much hormones. Having too much hormones can make your bodily functions speed up. You might experience fast heartbeats, lose weight quickly, and even begin to sweat a lot. Hyperthyroidism can be easily cured, but it can lead to serious complications if it is left alone.

Doctors may decide to place you under radioactive treatment. If this is the case, you will be asked to swallow liquids (or tablets) that contain radioactive iodide to control the damage in your thyroid glands. Often, more than one treatment is needed to restore a person's thyroid function.

Your symptoms should start to disappear after six to eight weeks of treatment, but you might still be required to continue taking medication for a year. It is also better if you continue to receive medical exams (to check whether the condition isn't slowly reemerging).

Doctors often recommend surgery for people under the age of 45, if their hypothyroidism is due to toxin exposure. That's because nodules tend to resist medication. Most hormone levels in the body return to normal once the surgery's completed.

Treatments for Subacute Thyroiditis

Subacute thyroditis is characterized as the inflammation of the thyroid. This condition can lead to temporary hyperthyroidism, which does not usually require medical intervention. The symptoms associated with the condition can easily be relieved by using acetaminophen. Doctors can also prescribe a powerful anti-inflammatory drug, such as prednisone, for a short period of time. However, remember that taking these drugs may create stomach ulcers, and even cause bone loss. Ask your doctor if you should take calcium supplements.

Treating Hypothyroidism

Hypothyroidism is a certain condition where the thyroid is not producing enough hormones. Women over the age of 60 are more susceptible to hypothyroidism. The condition causes an imbalance in the chemical reactions that occur within the body. It does not produce many symptoms, but it can lead to a number of health problems (like infertility, heart disease, and obesity).

Hypothyroidism requires a lifelong treatment, which involves thyroid replacement. So far, nothing can increase the production of hormones once it starts to slow down. That's why doctors often prescribe synthetic thyroid hormones, like levothyroxine, to hypothyroidism sufferers.

The Side effects of the drug include chest pain and nervousness. Adjusting your medication can help alleviate those side effects. Consult your doctor if you are taking other medications to ensure that they won't interfere with your thyroid treatment.

Treatment for Thyroid Cancer

Thyroid cancer is one of the most uncommon forms of cancer that is caused by the abnormal growth of cells in the thyroid glands. Most people with this type of cancer recover, since it is usually detected early and most treatments work well. However, the condition may return several years later. People who are usually exposed to radiation are also more at risk of developing thyroid cancer.

This type of cancer is usually treated by surgically removing the cancer tissue, or the whole thyroid gland. Any affected tissue around the thyroid will also be removed. After surgery, it can be treated using alternative therapy, which cleanses the body and restores immune function. It also balances hormone production.

Chapter 3:
Thyroid Diet Secrets

Almost 95% of thyroid problems happen when the autoimmune system of a person attacks the thyroid. This causes a number of complications since the body is confused by the sheer amount of hormones that end up being released.

Remember that no single food or drug can immediately cure your thyroid. However, you can start (as well as hasten) the healing process by adopting a holistic perspective, and following these suggestions:

- *Get enough Vitamin D*

  People who experience thyroid problems have low levels of Vitamin D. This vitamin is responsible for hormone production and thyroid function. The easiest way to get enough Vitamin D is by exposing yourself to the sun for 20 minutes (without using sunblock).

  Certain foods (such as salmon, sardines, and oysters) are also rich in Vitamin D. Vitamin D3 supplements can also help increase your Vitamin D levels.

- *Include fermented food*

  Fermented food can improve digestion, and strengthen your gut. This is particularly important in keeping your thyroid healthy. Inactive hormones are converted into active hormones in the liver and in the gut. These hormones drive weight changes and energy levels, as well as mental stability.

Fermented food provides the necessary bacteria that contribute to a healthy stomach. This also means that you will have more energy throughout the day. Some examples of fermented food include:

- *Miso soup.* A Japanese soup that is made of fermented soybeans and grains. It contains microorganisms that strengthens the body and improves stamina.

- *Kombucha.* This fermented black tea contains at least four to seven microorganisms.

- *Sauerkraut.* This fermented cabbage can also be good for your brain health. Eating this fermented food can also reduce anxiety and depression.

- *Pickles.* Pickles contain a great amount of probiotics. It is also one of the most popular fermented foods.

- *Coconut yogurt.* Eating coconut yogurt is a delicious way of getting both a probiotic boost and the enzymes needed for proper digestion.

- *Tempeh.* Tempeh contains proteins and amino acids. It is also one of the healthiest substitutes for bacon. You can eat it with vegetables, or add it to your sandwiches.

- *Kimchi.* Kimchi is a famous spicy Korean dish that is made from cabbage. It is said to increase energy and enhance digestion. It can also help clear the skin of impurities.

- *Get enough iron*

  Iron deficiency can contribute to thyroid problems. It is suggested that you take a blood test to determine if you lack iron. Symptoms of iron deficiency include anemia, tongue inflammation, and hair loss.

  Eat foods that are rich in iron (such as quinoa, beans, leafy greens, chia seeds,..). You can also take iron supplements, but be careful not to overdose yourself. Consume iron supplements together with vitamin C and E, since these vitamins help in the absorption of iron. Avoid mixing calcium and iron supplements together.

- *Identify your food sensitivities*

  Most people aren't aware that they have food sensitivities. Some of the most common food sensitivities involve soy, dairy, yeast, and nuts. One way of knowing if you have a certain food sensitivity is to try to eliminating one food from your diet and check whether you feel better afterwards. Once you reintroduce that food, you might experience headaches and feel fatigued. You'll also face acne-breakout risks. It is critical that you eliminate any food that triggers sensitivities.

- *Include good sources of proteins*

  You are encouraged to include different proteins in your diet. The key sources of protein are beans, lentils nuts, seeds and grains.

People with thyroid problem are often advised to consume high protein breakfasts, rather than eat carbohydrate-rich meals. This also reduces the risk of experiencing a sugar crash, and helps stabilize your glucose level throughout the day.

Remember that stable sugar levels are needed to maintain good thyroid health. If you currently suffer from any form of insulin resistance, consult your doctor before administering any thyroid medication or diet.

The suggested protein consumption for women is 46 grams, while men are advised to consume about 54 grams per day. One serving of salmon already contains 21 grams of protein while a cup of milk provides 8 grams.

- *Detox twice a year*

  The liver and the gut are responsible for the conversion of inactive hormones into energy. A healthy gut and liver is important in maintaining good thyroid health. Undergoing detox can provide a lot of relief for the body.

  It is best to follow detox diets during spring and autumn. Consult a holistic practitioner before starting any detox program. People suffering from hypoglycemia and insulin resistance should get medical advice.

- *Eat organic*

  The concept of eating organic food has been gaining popularity since naturally-grown eats are said to contain less toxins and pesticides. Chemicals, hormones, and synthetic fertilizers can compromise thyroid function.

Be aware that eating organic food does not necessarily mean that you need to spend money on expensive products. Try to get your produce at local markets and farms to save money.

- *Get fat*

Low fat levels can also lead to hormonal imbalance, which in turn affects the thyroid. However, be sure to consume healthy fat - excellent sources include butter, avocado, nuts (Almonds, Walnuts, Macadamias, etc), and seeds (Flax, Chia, Hemp, etc).

- *Be careful of goitrogens*

Goitrogens are foods that can interfere with your thyroid function. These foods include brussel sprouts, cauliflower, kale, broccoli, and turnip. This does not mean that you should totally eliminate these foods from your diet, but it is best to consume them in moderation.

- *Go for glutathione*

Glutathione is an antioxidant that can improve your immune system, and can boost your ability to regulate the immune system. It can also help heal the thyroid.

There foods that contain high amounts of glutathione are rare, but there are those that can increase the natural production of glutathione in the body. These foods include asparagus, peach, garlic, and grapefruit. The plant substances found in cabbages and cauliflowers can also replenish your glutathione levels.

- *Drink herbal teas*

  Drinking herbal teas is one of the best ways to increase thyroxin in the body. Black walnut tea contains iodine that stimulates the thyroid. Kelp and Irish moss tea can increase your metabolism, and improve the thyroid's hormone production capabilities.

- *Eat sea vegetables twice a week*

  Sea vegetables are a natural source of iodine, which support thyroid function. Incorporating sea vegetables into your diet can be simple. Just add kombu in a pot of beans, or sprinkle kelp granules in your salad. Nori wraps can also be used in different dishes.

- *Eat slowly*

  The thyroid gland is located at the throat. It connects the mind and body. When eat quickly, the food moves rapidly from your mouth down to your stomach. Eating slowly will enable the thyroid to properly "record" the food that is entering your body.

Chapter 4:
Foods to Avoid

Thyroid problems can be difficult to manage, but what you eat can greatly affect your treatment. Some nutrients can influence your thyroid function, while certain foods can inhibit the absorption of the necessary nutrients in your body. Here are some foods (and beverages) that you have to avoid:

- *Refined carbohydrates*

  Refined carbohydrates do not contain the necessary amount of nutrients needed for proper development. It is also a source of simple sugars. It can easily elevate your blood sugar levels, which could lead to sugar imbalances. Opt for whole fruits or whole grain carbohydrates as much as possible.

- *Avoid sugar*

  People who have hypothyroidism can experience fatigue and brain fog. This is usually caused by sugar. Sugar can be found in sweets, meat, and caffeinated drinks. These foods are also said to stress the thyroid gland, and thus can affect your blood sugar levels.

- *Processed foods*

  Processed foods in general are unhealthy and can cause inflammation. They also contain chemicals that can inhibit thyroid function and stop hormone conversion.

- *Juice and sodas*

  Sodas and juices are usually manufactured using fluoridated water, which can worsen thyroid problem. You should also avoid citrus-flavored sodas and drinks, since they contain bromine (a goitrogenic toxin).

- *Dairy*

  Try to limit the amount of dairy you consume. Some people who suffer from thyroid problems have food sensitivities that worsen certain symptoms. Eliminate these foods from your diet, and see whether you feel any better. Dairy also contains growth hormones and antibiotics, so go for organic ones as much as possible.

- *Get off the gluten*

  Gluten is a kind of protein that is often found in bread, pasta, and cake. Grains that are rich in gluten include wheat, barley, and rye. Gluten is known to inhibit immune system function, and can cause leaky gut syndrome (which lowers the body's defenses).

  Some studies show that most people with thyroid problems, such as hypothyroidism and hyperthyroidism, have gluten problems. Most patients report that they experience weight loss and see an increase in energy after removing gluten from their diet.

  Transitioning to a gluten-free diet may be challenging, but you do not have to commit to changes drastically. You can take gradual steps, such as making smoothies for breakfast rather than eating toast and butter. You can also find food substitutes (most stores have them).

Quinoa pasta, brown rice bread, and rice crackers are all delicious bread substitutes. You should also think about the potential benefits of going gluten free – such as losing weight, having more energy, experience fewer anxiety attacks, and being a lot less prone to depression. Try these treatments for two weeks, and record the changes that you'll feel.

- *Avoid soy products*

  Soy consumption has many advocates. People who experience thyroid problems, however, are most likely experiencing hormonal problems. That's why it's better to avoid soy, since it increases the levels of estrogen in the body. Fermented soy products (like tempeh or miso) can still be eaten, but try to avoid things like tofu, soy oil, and soymilk.

Chapter 5:
Herbal Remedies

Some people opt to try herbal remedies to cure their illnesses. After all, a holistic method is cheaper and safer than taking synthetic medications. Exercise and a healthy diet can also relieve your symptoms.

Here are some of herbs (which are most likely available in your natural food store) that can be used to improve your condition:

- *Cayenne*

  Cayenne can improve the circulation in the body. It also helps alleviate the symptoms caused by low thyroid hormone levels. It can hasten metabolism and boost your energy. It can also be used as a catalyst for other herbs, meaning that it increases the effectiveness of other herbal cures.

- *Ashwagandha root*

  This root is mostly used in Ayurvedic medicine. It can be classified as a Rasayana herb, which can improve your general health and can make you live longer. It also helps in maintaining proper thyroid function.

- *Kelp*

  Kelp is one of the most popular seaweeds, because it provides many benefits. It also contains a significant amount of iodine that stimulates your thyroid gland.

- *Myrrh*

  Myrrh is made from tree sap, and has a distinct odor. It can enhance thyroid function.

- *Coleus Forskohlii*

  Studies show that this herb can increase the secretion of thyroid hormones in the body. It also speeds up metabolism, while accelerating weight loss. It also supports good immune function.

- *Milk thistle*

  This herb is usually used to improve liver function, but it can also stimulate the thyroid gland. As an additional benefit, it can lower your cholesterol levels.

- *Black Cohosh*

  The black cohosh is a variety of the buttercup family. It can stimulate hormone production in the body. It also helps balance estrogen levels, thus ensuring optimal thyroid function.

Chapter 6:
Yoga Techniques

Thyroid problems can disrupt your blood's circulation. Performing the right exercise can ensure that blood is flowing correctly in your body. A 30-minute walk, or light aerobics, can improve your circulation. However, the best exercise for thyroid problems is yoga.

- *Easy pose and deep breathing*

  This is one of the easiest yoga poses. Sit with your legs crossed. Close your eyes, and start to breathe normally. Focus on taking deep breaths, and exhale through the mouth for ten seconds. Make sure that you do not stay in this position for too long.

- *Twisted seated pose*

  Sit on a mat with your legs crossed. Extend your arms on your sides. Inhale deeply and make sure that your spine is straight. Place your left hand on top of your right thigh, and twist your torso to the right. Hold the position for 30 seconds. Turn to the left, and place your right hand on your left leg. Hold for another 30 seconds.

- *Corpse pose*

  Lie on the floor and close your eyes. Relax and release any negative emotion and thought. Stand with your legs apart. Make sure that your legs are straight and firm. Cover your face with your hands. Take ten deep breaths. Lightly rub your face (using your hands), then take another ten breaths.

- *Bow pose*

Lie down, place your hands on your side, and place your palms on the ground. Bend your knees, and lift your heels near your buttocks. Grab your ankles. Shift your body weight towards your abdomen. Pull your ankles with your hands. Check whether your upper torso's rising (it should). Try to maintain your normal breathing pattern while doing the pose.

- *Mountain pose*

Stand with your feet apart. Place your arms at your sides, and keep your spine straight. Visualize a string that goes up to your spine and up to the sky. Pull your body straight. You can either bring your hands together in a prayer position, or leave them to your side.

- *Chair pose*

Start by doing the mountain pose, then bend your knees. Lower your buttocks to the floor. Imagine that you are sitting in an invisible chair. Try to go as low as you can. Bring your thighs up, until they're parallel to the ground. Lift your arms to lengthen your spine. Take ten deep breaths.

- *Warrior II pose*

Start with the mountain pose, then separate your legs. Make sure that your feet are about four feet apart.

Adjust accordingly, then bend your knee. Raise your arms to make it parallel to the floor. Turn the right foot towards the right side, and adjust your left foot for balance. Keep your torso straight. Your gaze should go beyond your hand. Take ten deep breaths, and repeat with the other side.

- *Triangle*

Maintain the wide stance from the Warrior II pose. Straighten your legs, but keep your arms raised. Stretch your upper body, and turn to the right. Raise your left arm over your head, and stretch towards the floor. Grab your ankle (or foot) if you need added support. Look at your left hand, and then hold the position for ten seconds.

- *Downward dos*

Lay your hand and feet to the ground. Curl your toes to ensure that they are in contact with the floor. Push your palms and feet. Straighten your legs, and lift your buttocks. Make sure that your back is flat, and your legs are straight. Keep your neck in neutral position (along with your spine), and keep the pose for 30 seconds.

- *Yoga lunge*

Start with the downward dog position, then step forward. Place your right foot forward, and afterwards put it between your hands. Arch your back, and look at the ceiling. Move your palms to the floor, and then hold the position for ten seconds. Push back to a downward dog position. Switch to the other side, and repeat.

- *Pigeon*

  Come to your knees, and then swing your foot forward. Your knees should be between your hands. Slide your left leg and try to extend it straight without straining your groin. Arch your back, and hold the position for ten seconds – release, and then lower your head to the floor. Hold for another ten seconds before switching to another position.

- *Extended triangle pose*

  This is considered as one of the foundation poses. It is a great stress reliever, and can be a good stretching exercise. It can also improve your digestion and alleviate anxiety. Stand with your feet apart. Gently lean to one side, and stretch your arms. Place one hand to your knees, while stretching the other above your head. Hold the position for ten seconds before releasing.

- *Shoulder stand*

  This is one of the advanced yoga poses. Do this with caution. People who have never tried this position may practice by placing their legs up to the wall. Start by lying on your back, and then bring your feet close to your buttocks. Use your core to lift your feet off the floor. Your legs should be pointing to the sky. You chin should be close to your chest. Look at your navel (remember to engage your abdomen). Use your hands to support your lower back. Stay in the position for as long as you'd like.

- *Eagle pose*

  This active and empowering pose can help relieve stress and release negative energy. The eagle pose can also improve your balance and circulation. Imagine sitting in an invisible chair. Place both hands in front of you. Place your left elbow on top of your right forearm, and twist your right arm around your left arm. Keep your left foot firmly planted on the ground. Lift your right leg then rest it on top of your left thigh. Twist your leg so that your right foot is resting at the back of your left leg.

- *Standing forward bend*

  This pose is often used to transition from one pose to another. This posture stretches the hamstrings, hips, and legs. You could keep your legs either straight or slightly bent. Place your palms next to your feet.

- *Savasana*

  This is a good pose to end your exercise. You can place a small pillow between your knees for extra comfort. Lie on your back and keep your feet apart. Place your arms to the side.

  Relax your body, and think about releasing all your stress. Let go of the tension through your extremities. Take your time, and take as many breaths as you like.

Chapter 7:
Other Types of Common Thyroid Disorders

Thyroid is a gland located just below the Adam's apple. This small gland controls hormones in the body that is responsible for your metabolism. Unfortunately, there is more than one type of thyroid disorder. Here are the most common types of thyroid disorders:

Hashimoto's Disease

Hashimoto's Disease is also called lymphatic thyroiditis. It is caused by an underactive thyroid. While Hashimoto's disease can affect any age group, it is more common among middle-aged women.

Hashimoto's disease develops when the thyroid gland is unable to produce hormones properly because the immune system inhibits its function.

Symptoms:

Early stages of the disease do not present recognizable symptoms. It can also develop slowly for several years before being diagnosed.

- Depression

- Irregular menstruation

- Fatigue and sleepiness

- Constipation

- Mild weight gain

- Cold intolerance

Diagnosis:

Testing for thyroid hormones is the first step in treating the disorder. Once the doctor confirms that the patient is suffering from the symptoms of Hashimoto's disease, he might even consider using a blood test and see if there is any form of thyroid deficiency. The blood test can confirm any abnormalities in the production of antibodies.

Treatment:

Most patients are prescribed with medication that can increase hormone levels. Since the disease develops slowly and can be detected early, it's not that difficult to treat and most patients have high recovery rates.

Graves' Disease

Graves' disease is usually the cause of hypothyroidism or the overproduction of hormones. Since thyroid hormones affect the whole body, any symptom of the disease can have significant impact on the patient's overall wellbeing. Graves' disease can be inherited. Any age group can develop Grave's disease but it is more common among women under the age of 40.

Symptoms:

Grave's disease is similar to hypothyroidism that it also results to an increased amount of hormones in the blood. The symptoms below aren't associated with the disease alone and can also be triggered by other conditions.

- Difficulty sleeping

- Anxiety and fatigue

- Altered menstrual cycle

- Fast heartbeat

- Enlarged thyroid

- Bulging eyes

- Excessive sweating

Diagnosis:

The doctor can usually detect physical symptoms like enlarged thyroid, rapid pulse, light sensitivity and bulging eyes. A blood test can also show low amount of thyroid hormones which can indicate Graves' disease.

Patients may also undergo a test to measure their iodine uptake to see how fast they can absorb iodine in their system. Fast absorption of iodine can be indicative of Grave's disease.

Treatment:

There is still no cure for Grave's disease. Modern science has yet to find a way to prevent the immune system from mistakenly destroying the thyroid.

The treatment for Graves's is focused on managing the symptoms of the disease and stopping the overproduction of hormones. Some doctors prescribe Beta blockers used for anxiety and irregular heartbeat.

Anti-thyroid medicines can also be used to limit the amount of hormones produced by the thyroid. You can also try radioactive iodine therapy that is administered through the mouth. The radioiodine destroys the thyroid cells and renders it incapable of producing hormones. The doctor can also permanently remove the thyroid through surgery. However, this is usually seen as a last resort since patients will need hormonal replacement for the rest of their lives after the surgery.

Graves' disease can cause complications and even thyrotoxic crisis that can drastically worsen the symptoms. Fortunately, the disease can be detected early and most treatments have a high rate of success.

Goiter

Goiter can be described as the abnormal enlargement of the thyroid. It is usually caused by iodine deficiency. It can also be triggered by hypothyroidism. Anyone can be affected by goiter but it is most common in regions without iodine-rich food. Other factors can also cause goiter such as medicine and radiation exposure; pregnancy can also increase the risk of developing goiter.

Symptoms:

Goiter is usually painless but the enlarged goiter can make it difficult for patients to breathe or swallow. These are some classic signs of goiter:

- Enlargement of the neck

- Coughing

- Difficulty swallowing

- Hoarseness

Diagnosis:

The doctor may ask the patient to swallow in order to know if the patient experiences difficulty in swallowing. Blood tests results can show any abnormal levels of hormones. An ultrasound can also confirm the presence of any nodules or swelling in the neck.

Treatment:

The treatment for goiter depends on the size of the thyroid. Goiter caused by iodine deficiency can be treated with small amounts of iodine. Patients can also try radioactive iodine.

Goiter can also be associated with other thyroid disorder like Graves' disease. Goiter itself is benign. Sometimes goiter can even disappear on its own but it can also grow bigger and cause serious complications.

Thyroid Nodules

Thyroid nodules grow on or inside the thyroid. The lumps can be solid or it can also be filled with fluid. Majority of the nodules are painless and harmless. It is only in rare cases where these nodules become cancerous. Women are more prone to developing thyroid nodules than men. The risk of developing nodules increases with age.

Symptoms:

Thyroid symptoms can be confused with those of other diseases. Most of the symptoms are not severe but some of the lumps can become so large that they cause difficulty in breathing and swallowing. Some of the nodules can also produce hormones that can disturb the balance in the system.

- Nervousness

- Increased appetite

- Increased pulse rate

- Sweaty skin

- Weight loss

Thyroid nodules triggered by Hashimoto's disease will have similar symptoms to hypothyroidism.

- Weight gain

- Thinning hair

- Fatigue

- Cold intolerance

- Flakey and dry skin

Diagnosis:

The nodules are usually detected during physical examination. They can also be detected in an ultrasound and CT scan. Doctors can carry out fine-needle biopsy to take sample cells from the nodules to determine if they're cancerous.

Treatment:

Benign nodules are rarely life threatening and usually do not need treatment. For benign biopsy, treatment may include radioactive iodine and hormone suppression. Cancerous nodules are usually rare but are treated by removing the thyroid through surgery. Radiation surgery is also possible. Chemotherapy is required if the cancer already spread to the other parts of the body.

Chapter 8:
Exercise and Thyroid Problems

Certain health conditions, like thyroid disease, can make it difficult to commit to an active lifestyle. Since the thyroid is responsible for regulating hormones that control your metabolism, thyroid problems can impair your ability to exercise. However, it is a known fact that exercise is an essential part of a healthy lifestyle. Understanding your thyroid problem can help you look for ways to integrate exercise into your daily routine.

Hypothyroidism's effect on exercise

The risk of acquiring hypothyroidism increases with age. An impaired thyroid can affect your body functions. Most people do not feel the symptoms of hypothyroidism until the disease progresses. One of the first signs of hypothyroidism is feeling fatigued during physical activities. Patients may also notice that they feel sluggish and they might gain weight despite normal diet and exercise.

Exercise for Hypothyroidism

Regular workouts can already be challenging for people with hypothyroidism. Since hypothyroidism slows metabolism, patients are prone to unwanted weight gain. Their cholesterol levels can also be high and they may suffer from cognitive impairment. Regular exercise can be a good part of the treatment plan and help people manage the symptoms.

Regular aerobic exercise improves cholesterol levels and helps people burn excess fat. Exercise can also help improve mental health. Both aerobic exercise and weight training can improve cognitive function and reduce anxiety. Exercise can also reduce the risk of stroke, cancer, stress and diabetes.

Best Exercise for Hypothyroidism

Doctors usually recommend both aerobic exercise and weight training. Aerobic exercise, like jogging, walking, cycling and swimming, can improve your overall health and help burn fat in the process.

You should aim for moderate intensity workouts like water aerobics, playing sports and dancing. After you have gained enough endurance, you can increase the intensity and try running and playing vigorous sports.

Weight training should be a part of your treatment to help build muscle and to keep your metabolism active throughout the day. Strength training is very important especially when the patient does not take any medication and metabolism starts to decrease significantly.

Do at least two days of strength training each week and make sure to let your muscles rest in between sessions. You can try lifting weights or using resistance bands. Bodyweight workouts like push-ups and squats are also beneficial.

Before you start your exercise regimen, make sure that you speak to your doctor about it. It is also important that you start slowly. Gradually increase your routine's intensity as you become more comfortable with physical exertion.

Hyperthyroidism's Effect on Exercise

Hyperthyroidism occurs when the thyroid produces too much hormones and increases your metabolic process drastically.

Hyperthyroidism can make your heart beat faster which makes it difficult for you to exercise. Any activity that raises heart rate, which is already too high, can lead to exercise intolerance.

One symptom of overactive thyroid is unintentional weight loss which can also cause weakness and fatigue. Patients may also experience intolerance for extreme exercise and sweat more than usual even when at rest.

Exercise for Hyperthyroidism

An overactive thyroid can make it much more challenging to exercise. Patients with hyperthyroidism can combine diet, medication and exercise to manage their symptoms. Less vigorous exercises are greatly recommended for people with hyperthyroidism. Thyroid problems are usually linked to osteoporosis, which reduces the density of your bones. A healthy lifestyle, which includes a healthy diet, calcium supplements and weight exercises, can be beneficial.

Best Exercise for Hyperthyroidism

General exercise is recommended for people with hyperthyroid disease. You can do 30 to 60 minutes of aerobic exercise every day. The most recommended aerobic exercise includes activities that can engage your large muscle. These activities include biking, swimming and dancing.

Resistance and strength exercise can be more manageable for people with hyperthyroidism since it does not increase your heart rate much. Aim to do resistance training two to three times in a week with at least 48 hours of rest in between. Weight bearing exercise like heavy gardening and mowing can also help strengthen the bones and prevent osteoporosis.

Some doctors also recommend yoga, meditation and Tai Chi for people with hyperthyroidism. These are gentle enough not to spike your heart rate too much but can still give you the full benefits of a workout. Yoga, meditation and Tai Chi are also especially effective in reducing stress and anxiety.

Chapter 9:
Adrenal Stress and Thyroid

Stress can be debilitating for anyone. Harmful effects of stress on the adrenals can also affect your thyroid health. Adrenals are walnut shaped glands located above the kidneys. These organs secrete hormones like norepinephrine, cortisol and epinephrine. These hormones are also responsible for regulating stress response. These hormones are linked to the thyroid glands. In fact, healthy adrenal glands can help the thyroid function better.

Most people are aware of the symptoms of stress like mood swings and sleep disturbance. However, there are more serious symptoms of stress that can also place burden on the adrenals. The symptoms include food intolerance, blood sugar fluctuation and gut dysfunction.

These symptoms cause the adrenals to produce more stress hormones, causing an imbalance in the body. Adrenal stress is one of the most common problems people have to deal with.

Weak adrenals can trigger hypothyroid symptoms even if there isn't any problem with the thyroid itself. In this case, thyroid treatment becomes ineffective and unnecessary. The best way to combat this is to address the adrenal problem to improve thyroid function.

The most indirect effect of adrenals to the thyroid is their influence on blood sugar. Cortisol imbalance can cause hyperglycemia or hypoglycemia, which can trigger hypothyroid symptoms.

Here are the direct impacts of adrenal stress on thyroid function:

- *Adrenal Stress Disrupts the HPA Axis*

HPA axis or the hypothalamic pituitary adrenal axis is a network of interactions in the hypothalamus, adrenal glands and pituitary gland. This axis helps regulate body temperature, immune system, sexuality and even digestion. It also controls the body's response to trauma. Studies show that adrenal stress can reduce pituitary and hypothalamic function. Since these organs can affect hormone production, it can also affect and suppress thyroid function.

Inflammatory cytokines released during stress can also affect the HPA axis and reduce thyroid hormones.

- *Adrenal stress reduces the conversion of T4 to T3*

94% of the hormones produced by the thyroid are T4. However, this cannot be used by the cells, so it has to be converted to T3 before being absorbed by the body. The inflammatory cytokines can also reduce the amount of T4 being converted to T3.

- *Adrenal stress promotes autoimmunity and weakens immune barriers*

The GI tract is one of the body's primary immune barriers. It can protect the internal system from foreign substances. Adrenal stress weakens the immune system in general. Weak immune system means that large proteins and antigens get into the bloodstream and brain. Being exposed to these agents can increase your risk of developing autoimmune diseases like Hashimoto's.

- *Adrenals stress causes thyroid resistance*

Thyroid hormones need to activate receptors in the cells before it can work. Inflammatory cytokines can suppress the thyroid function and reduce sensitivity of the receptors. It is the same as insulin resistance where the cells lose their ability to respond to insulin.

This is apparent to conditions like Hashimoto's disease where the patient is taking replacement hormones but still continues to suffer from hypothyroid symptoms. In this case, inflammation reduces thyroid receptor sensitivity and triggers symptoms of thyroid problem even if all hormone levels appear normal.

- *Adrenal stress causes hormonal imbalance*

Cortisol is produced by the adrenals during stressful situations. High cortisol levels can trigger chronic stress and reduce the liver's ability to remove any excess estrogen from the bloodstream.

Excess estrogen levels can increase the production of thyroid-binding globulin. These are the proteins that hormones attach to as they are being transported throughout the body.

Thyroid hormone is inactive if it is still bound to the TBG. It must detach from the TBG before it can activate any receptor. High levels of TBG decrease the percentage of free thyroid hormones. Aside from adrenal stress, elevated levels of TBG are also caused by birth control pills and estrogen replacements.

How to Balance Your Adrenals

Adrenal stress is almost always caused by another condition. It can be triggered by gut inflammation, anemia and even blood sugar spikes. These conditions should also be addressed directly or else any form of treatment for the adrenals will become useless. Here are some guidelines in keeping your adrenals healthy:

- *Diet and Nutrition*

The goal is to eliminate any food that can increase your blood sugar level, like sugar, alcohol and caffeine. However, removing substances that you are used to, like coffee, can also be stressful for your adrenals; so, try to minimize your consumption gradually.

- *Sleep*

Staying up late and not getting enough sleep can be stressful for your adrenal glands. Remember that the adrenal glands are being repaired while you are sleeping. Resting as much as you need for is not being lazy or selfish. It is a crucial part of a healthy lifestyle and helps you recover faster.

Also, do not depend on coffee and sleeping pills to regulate your sleeping pattern. Depending on these substances can counter act your circadian rhythm and may be doing more harm than good. The solution to feeling awake in the morning is not coffee but to have enough sleep. Magnesium supplements can relax you and help you fall asleep better. Those can also support your adrenal function.

- *Stress Reduction*

Identify situations, relationships and people that bring you high levels of stress. If you have been suffering from stress for a while, it can be helpful to make a list of your stress triggers. This can help you eliminate any unnecessary stress from your life. Also, give yourself some time to relax and unwind.

Reduce your exposure to chemicals like fluoride, chlorine and other endocrine disruptors since they can be contributing to your stress. Moderate physical activity is also recommended over fast-paced aerobic workout if you are trying to keep your adrenals stress free.

Chapter 10:
Blood Sugar and Thyroid Function

The American Association of Clinical Endocrinologist says that almost 27 million Americans suffer from thyroid problems. Half of these cases are undiagnosed. Metabolic syndrome and insulin resistance are also becoming more common and are listed as two of the top causes of death in the developed world.

Studies show that there is a connection between thyroid problems and metabolic syndrome. Diabetics have greater risks of developing thyroid disorders, while people with thyroid disorders have high chances of developing metabolic syndromes.

Thyroid function is largely regulated by keeping the blood sugar level normal and keeping a normal blood sugar depends on a healthy thyroid function.

High blood sugar effect on thyroid

Metabolic syndrome can be defined as a group of metabolic risk factors appearing together like abdominal obesity, insulin resistance, inflammation, high blood pressure, high cholesterol level and tendency to form blood clots.

Metabolic syndrome is caused by consuming too many carbohydrates. This is why some people call metabolic syndrome as 'excess carbohydrate disease'. Eating too many carbohydrates triggers the pancreas to secrete insulin to move the glucose from the blood into the cells. However, the cells lose their ability to respond to insulin over time. The pancreas produces more insulin to try to get the glucose into the cells, leading to insulin resistance.

Studies show that insulin surges can lead to the destruction of thyroid gland for people suffering from autoimmune disease.

Low blood sugars effect on thyroid

Low blood sugar can also cause problems for the thyroid just as much as high blood sugar. The body is programmed to treat low blood sugar as a threat for survival. Prolonged hypoglycemia or low blood sugar level can trigger seizure, coma and death.

If the blood sugar level is lower than normal, the adrenal glands secrete more hormones called the cortisol. This hormone triggers the liver to increase glucose production to bring blood sugar back to normal levels.

However, cortisol is also involved in a genetic human response known as 'flight or fight'. This leads to an increase in heart rate and lung action. The blood vessels in the muscles also expand in preparation for action. Constant cortisol release due to low blood sugar can affect pituitary function and without a properly functioning pituitary gland, the thyroid cannot function well.

Some people can suffer from both hyperglycemia and hypoglycemia. This condition is known as dysglycemia. Dysglycemia inflames the gut, brain and lungs. It also causes hormonal imbalance and disrupts the normal detoxification process. Any treatment for your thyroid will be ineffective if you do not treat dysglycemia as well.

Thyroid effect on blood sugar

In a reverse situation, thyroid problems can also cause metabolic syndrome and even dysglycemia. It presents several symptoms including slow rate of glucose uptake, slow clearance of insulin from blood, slow absorption of glucose and slow response of insulin.

These symptoms may be diagnosed as hypoglycemia. People who are hypothyroid do not respond well to glucose. This means that even if they have normal blood sugar levels, they still experience symptoms of hypoglycemia including headache, irritability and hunger. Since the cells are not getting enough glucose, the body releases more cortisol and triggers a chronic stress response.

Measuring blood sugar levels

It is important to know whether you have low or high blood sugar. There are two factors to consider when trying to keep your blood sugar normal – fasting blood glucose and post-prandial blood glucose.

Fasting blood glucose is the method of measuring your blood sugar in the morning before your eat or drink anything. The normal fasting blood glucose is between 75-95 mg/dL.

During the 90's, fasting blood sugar levels is believed to indicate future diabetic cases. Although 80 mg/dL is often the cut off, some people can dip as low as 70 mg/dL especially if they follow a low carbohydrate diet.

The post-prandial blood sugar is measured one or two hours after eating. The normal range is 120 mg/dL. If you are hypoglycemic, you will need to keep your sugar level above 75 during the day. You can do this by following a low to moderate carbohydrate diet and eat frequent meals to ensure that you have enough energy supply.

If you are hyperglycemic, you will need to keep your blood sugar level below 120 after eating. The only way to successfully do this is to limit the amount of carbohydrates you eat.

It can be challenging to measure just how much carbohydrates you need to consume during the day. Using a blood glucose meter and testing your blood sugar level few times in the day can help you identify your limits. A blood glucose meter can be the simplest, most cost effective tool that you can use to know just how much carbohydrates you need.

Tips in Keeping Your Blood Sugar Stable

You can do small things every day to prevent spikes and dips in your blood sugar. Rather than merely focusing on the foods that you shouldn't eat, you should also try to explore other foods that you can add into your diet.

- *Nuts*

Nuts like pistachios, walnuts and almonds contain healthy fat that slow down the absorption of sugar into the blood system. However, make sure that you also eat nuts in moderation, especially if you are trying to keep your weight in check. Remember that even healthy fats contain calories.

- *Consume whole grains*

Whole grains food are rich in fiber and contain beta glucan. This is a soluble fiber that can slow down the process of emptying your stomach and prevent sugar spikes. Remember that whole grains are still carbohydrates and can also raise your blood sugar, although not as quickly as processed and refined foods can. Substitute whole grains for refined variety instead.

- *Be versatile in using vinegar*

A study published in a medical journal suggests that vinegar can slow the absorption of sugar in your body. The study suggests that consuming 2 ounces of apple cider vinegar can improve your blood sugar levels.

- *Do not skip meals*

People who are suffering from blood sugar imbalance should never skip their meals. Consuming more food in just one or two meals can trigger blood sugar fluctuations. A regular diet of three main meals with two snacks can help maintain healthy blood sugar levels.

- *Avoid drinking alcohol on an empty stomach*

Drinking alcohol on an empty stomach triggers a drop in blood sugar levels 24 hours later. This occurs as your body is trying to remove the alcohol in your system. It is very important to eat before you drink any alcoholic beverage. You also have to be careful since some symptoms of low blood sugar can be mistaken for drunkenness.

- *Make sure to plan ahead*

Carrying healthy snacks with you all the time can prevent you from skipping meals and letting your blood sugar go too low. You can also carry quick acting-glucose tablets to keep your sugar level in check.

Chapter 11:
Gut Health and Thyroid Function

Poor gut health has been linked to several chronic conditions. Poor gut health can cause several thyroid disease like Hashimoto's disease. Low thyroid function can also lead to inflammation and leaky gut syndrome.

Why the gut is so important

The gut contains trillions of bacteria that are responsible for food digestion and providing nutrients. Every food and drink that you consume can affect your gut heath.

It is important to maintain a healthy balance of bacteria in your gut. If you have 80% good bacteria and 20% bad bacteria, you would feel energized and nimble. Having a healthy balance also ensures that bacteria can do their job properly and can keep the bad bacteria in check.

However if there is an overgrowth of bad bacteria, it can cause a lot of health problems for you. Bad bacteria buildup can lead to inflammation, allergy, headache, and autoimmune disease.

There are a lot of factors that can affect the balance between good and bad bacteria. Medication like antibiotics, toxins chemicals and even stress can reduce good bacteria in your gut and gives the bad bacteria an advantage.

The food you consume can play a role in keeping a healthy ratio of good and bad bacteria. The food is processed and either absorbed by the body or passed into the gut. The gut digests the food further and extracts the nutrients, minerals and vitamins.

It is said the gut functions as the second brain of the body. The gut has around 100 million neurons in the intestines which transmits information throughout the body. It can also control your digestion and send information to the brain about the status of your gut health.

The connection between gut and thyroid health

The gut is a tube that passes through the mouth to the anus. Any substance that passes in the mouth without being digested passes out to the other end. One of the most important functions of the gut is to keep foreign substance from entering the system. Another function of the gut is to host 70% of the immune tissues.

The immune system in the gut is referred to as GALT or gut associated lymphoid tissue. It's also composed of several tissues that store immune cells. These cells include T & B lymphocytes that can produce enough antibodies to fight off infection.

Problems can occur if the gut is compromised and the barriers of the intestines are breached. Large protein enters into the bloodstream and the immune system attacks it. Studies show that this immune response can trigger the development of autoimmune disease like Hashimoto's.

Thyroid hormones can also affect the junctions in the stomach and intestines. These junctions form the protective barrier of the gut. T3 and T4 protect this lining and prevent ulcer formation.

Gut bacteria and thyroid connection

Gut bacteria can help covert inactive T4 hormone to the active T3. In fact, almost 20% of T4 is converted in the gastrointestinal tract. Healthy gut bacteria produce intestinal sulfates that are responsible for converting T4. Any imbalance in healthy gut bacteria reduces the levels of T3. This is the reason why some people can have poor gut health and experience thyroid problems despite having normal hormone lab results.

Inflammation can also affect the conversion of T3 and increase the levels of cortisol in the system. Studies also show that intestinal bacteria can affect thyroid metabolism by reducing the hormone levels, making the hormones insensitive and promoting autoimmune thyroid disease.

Other gut and thyroid connections

Low stomach acid increases the risk of the intestines being invaded by bacteria. This makes it more prone to inflammation and infection. Constipation can also hinder hormonal function and increase estrogen levels. Low thyroid function can lead to constipation and malabsorption.

Keeping a healthy gut

The connection between the gut and the thyroid is easy to establish. This leads to the conclusion that people with thyroid problems need to take care of their gut health more to prevent and stop thyroid problem symptoms.

Tips in Keeping Your Gut Healthy

Since digestive issues can have a huge impact on a person's strength and vitality, keeping your gut healthy can be one of the best things that you can do to improve your overall health.

You need to do two things to keep your gut healthy – eat a lot of plant-based and nutrient-rich food, as well as maintain a healthy lifestyle.

- *Probiotic supplements*

Taking probiotic supplements is one of the best things that you can do for your digestive tract. It can increase the number of good bacteria in your gut and improve your immune system in the process. This can also help relieve any digestive issues that you may experience. It becomes more important to take probiotic supplements if you are taking antibiotics since it can kill even the good bacteria.

If your symptoms persist despite taking probiotic supplements, you may want to try other remedies like herbal antibiotics that can kill excess bad bacteria. You can also take a glutamine formula that can repair your intestinal linings. This can increase your digestive enzymes to help your stomach digest the food better.

- *Eat probiotic foods*

Fermented food that contains good bacteria has been proven to be beneficial for your gut health. Fermented foods like miso, kefir, kimchi and sauerkraut can be a good addition to your diet. Avoid vinegar-based fermented food since this can kill good bacteria.

- *Eat prebiotic whole foods*

Certain foods can also promote the growth of good bacteria. Plant-based foods that are rich in fiber can support your gut health. Foods like garlic, onions, artichokes and bananas are good prebiotic foods.

- *Eat regularly but not constantly*

Make sure that you give your gut enough time to clean excess waste and bacteria. The muscles in the intestines move every 90 minutes to two hours but it is interrupted when you eat. This means that constant snacking can slow down your digestion and lead to bacterial overgrowth. This does not mean that you have to go through long periods without eating but you also have to make sure that you are giving your gut enough time to perform their job.

- *Stay hydrated*

As a general rule, you should drink half of your bodyweight in ounces each day. So if you are 130 pounds, you should aim to consume 65 oz of water. Your gut needs enough water to move the waste through your system. It also prevents bloating and constipation. Being dehydrated increases your risk of suffering from bacterial overgrowth and inflammation.

- *Eat less sugar and refined foods*

Sugar is food for bad bacteria. Eating processed and sugar rich food can derail your efforts of balancing good and bad bacteria in your system. Most people find it difficult to quit eating sugar and processed foods because these can be addictive. You can perform a sugar detox to help reset your taste buds.

- *Reduce stress*

Chronic stress can trigger a fight or flight response and cause your digestion to slow down. The muscles that push the waste in your system freezes and digestive enzymes decrease. Make sure that you are coping with stress by spending some quiet time alone and doing some exercises like meditation, yoga and even breathing therapy.

Chapter 12:
Common Treatments for Thyroid Problems

Thyroid disorders that are caused by under or over production of hormones can be successfully managed with conventional and alternative treatment. Natural remedies as well as clinical drugs can offer relief from discomfort and help restore the balance of hormones.

Conventional treatment includes prescription drugs while alternative remedies involve incorporating food, herbs, and exercises to help reduce symptoms. Make sure that you undergo medical evaluation before starting any form of treatment regimen.

Conventional Treatment

The most common treatments for thyroid problems include radioactive iodine treatment, medication and surgery.

If your doctor suggests the radioactive treatment, you will be asked to swallow a liquid or tablet that contains iodine to damage the cells of the thyroid gland and inhibit their ability to produce hormones. In some cases, more than one treatment is needed to restore proper hormonal balance. Be warned that patients can also develop hypothyroidism as a result of this.

If you opt for thyroid medication, your symptoms should start to disappear in six to eight weeks. Patients are usually advised to keep on taking the medication for one year. Your doctor will need to follow up on the condition every few months to see if the medication can be stopped.

Surgery is often seen as last resort, especially for people who cannot take anti-thyroid medicine and people with large and cancerous nodules.

Some thyroid conditions, like subacute thyroiditis, can cause hyperthyroidism symptoms but may not need any form of treatment. Thyroid pain can be relieved by taking acetaminophen, like Anacin or Tylenol. People can also opt to take aspirin but you should not give them to children and teens under the age of 19 since they can increase the risk of Reye Syndrome.

Doctors can prescribe a stronger medicine, like prednisone or dexamethasone. These are potent anti-inflammatory drugs that should only be used for a short period.

People with hypothyroidism need to use thyroid replacement their entire life. Most aggressive treatments render the thyroid completely non-functional so patients need to get their hormones from something else. Doctors usually prescribe levothyroxine which is a synthetic thyroid hormone.

Side effects of these drugs include chest pain and nervousness. Drug dosage can be adjusted to suit the patient and to alleviate some side effects. Make sure that you inform your doctor if you are taking other drugs like estrogens, antidepressants, heart disease medications, and blood thinning drugs.

In cases of thyroid cancer, surgery is usually seen as the best option to remove the cancerous tissue. If the cancer has already spread to other organs and tissues, it should also be removed.

Natural Treatment

Following a healthy lifestyle can increase your chances of recovery dramatically. Some people also opt to use natural treatment first before they try more aggressive procedures. Some aspects of a healthy lifestyle, like diet and applicable exercise, have already been explored in the first parts of the book. Here are some general guidelines in keeping your thyroid healthy, making it easier to manage symptoms:

For hypothyroid:

- *More iodine*

The two main causes of low thyroid hormone production are aging and iodine deficiency. In modern times, most people need to restrict their sodium intake. Medicine like antihistamines and anti-depressants can also affect and slow the thyroid function. Make sure that you are getting enough iodine from your diet.

- *Avoid Goitrogens*

Goitrogens are food that can interfere with the thyroid process and lead to low hormone production most especially if they are consumed raw. Cooking goitrogen foods can render their anti-thyroid properties ineffective. The most common goitrogen are vegetables from the broccoli family, including cauliflower and cabbage. Other goitrogens include kale, corn, mustard, spinach, radish, watercress, pine nuts, millet, pears, almonds, rutabaga and soybeans.

- *Regular Exercise*

Boost your thyroid function through exercise. Working out for 40 minutes, three times a day, can help improve overall health. Yoga can also help calm you and reduce stress.

- *Get enough Vitamin D*

Enough levels of Vitamin D can improve the body's immunity and increase calcium absorption.

For Hyperthyroid:

- *Consume goitrogenic foods*

What may be bad for one condition can be good for the other. Goitrogenic foods can help people with hyperthyroid since these inhibit the production of hormones.

- *Maintain balanced nutrition and ensure enough vitamin and mineral intake*

People with hyperthyroid should make sure that they have enough nutrients to offset their high metabolic activity. If you follow a relatively healthy diet, you are already getting enough vitamins and minerals. Avoid diuretic beverage that can remove nutrients from your body.

An overactive thyroid can make you zinc deficient and may also affect the metabolism of calcium in your body. Make sure that you increase your consumption of zinc and calcium. Vitamins high in antioxidants, such as Vitamin C, E and A, can also help manage hyperthyroid conditions.

- *Try herbs*

The most effective herbs for hyperthyroidism include eleuthero, bugleweed and motherwort. Eleuthero can strengthen weak adrenals and prevent autoimmune disease the Graves' disease. Bugleweed can manage the symptoms of hyperthyroidism well. However, make sure that bugleweed is not consumed by a person with hypothyroidism. Motherwort is an herb that can reduce palpitations and other symptoms.

Self-Acupuncture for thyroid problems

Self-acupuncture can help with both hyperthyroidism and hypothyroidism. Stimulating the thyroid pressure points can help restore the natural hormonal balance in your body. The thyroid pressure points in the body include the base of your throat, chest and neck.

Chapter 13:
Interpreting Thyroid Results

Test results are crucial in diagnosing thyroid problems and determining the appropriate treatment for patients. It can be confusing to discuss your test results with your doctor if you have no medical background. There are a lot of factors to consider when interpreting thyroid test results but knowing the basics can greatly help you.

Blood Tests

Blood tests are usually done for patients who suspect that they have thyroid problems. Learning how to interpret your own thyroid results can help you to understand the treatment that your doctor might be proposing to you.

- *TSH test*

The TSH or thyroid stimulating hormone is measured in the bloodstream to determine thyroid problems. It is also called as the thyrotropin stimulating hormone test. If the TSH level is elevated, it indicates hypothyroidism. If the test results show lower than normal, then it is usually indicative of hyperthyroidism.

Doctors can follow the old or new standard in determining the normal range. In 2003, the American Association of Clinical Endocrinologist changed the normal TSH range between 0.3 and 3.0. The old standard is a little higher at 0.5 to 5.5. There is still an ongoing debate about these ranges and some doctors may follow the older or the newer standard. Make sure to ask your doctor about this.

- *Free Thyroxine*

Free Thyroxine or Free T4 is a test that measures the thyroxin in the bloodstream. Elevated levels indicate hypothyroidism while suppressed levels can indicate hypothyroidism.

Free thyroixine in the blood represents the hormones that are available for use and can be absorbed by the cells. Bound thyroxine are those that are still circulating in the bloodstream but may not be available for immediately because it is affected by other factors like pregnancy, disease or drugs. Since free thyroxine is immediately available, they are seen as better gauge of the hormonal status of patients.

- *Total T4/ Serum Thyroxine*

This is a test that measures the total amount of thyroxine in the blood. The total amount of thyroixine in the body can be affected by different factors like estrogen states and even pregnancy.

- *Total T3/ Total Triiodothyronine*

T3 is a thyroid hormone that is usually elevated in cases of hyperthyroidism and suppressed when a person has hypothyroidism.

- *Free T3/Free Triiodothyonine*

This test measures the unbound levels of triiodothyonine in the blood and does not include T3 that is not available for use.

- *RT3/ reverse T3*

RT3 is a controversial test in thyroid treatment. Some doctors do not consider this test in diagnosing thyroid problems while others believe that it is essential in maintaining hormonal balance in the body.

RT3 is a metabolite of thyroixine. When the T4 loses its iodine compound, it becomes T3 which is an active thyroid hormone. However, the body is also capable of converting T4 instead of RT3.

Conventional endocrinologist believes that a person's T4 and T3 levels function seamlessly and it does not indicate thyroid dysfunction. However, hormone experts believe that an increase of RT3 levels in the blood can reflect cellular hypothyroidism.

RT3 is an antithyroid that can stimulate the metabolic process. Reverse T3 binds to the receptors and sticks to it but nothing happen so it blocks the thyroid function. It can also be defined as a hibernation hormone that can be triggered by stress and disease. It affects the body by lowering the metabolism. This means that even though a person may have normal thyroid levels but if their RT3 results are high, they are actually suffering from hypothyroidism.

One of the ways to address high RT3 levels is through medication that contains T3. In some cases, this medication is prescribed as a separate treatment for thyroid problems. However, it can also be added to synthetic T4 prescription drugs.

The main challenge in addressing RT3 is finding a doctor who is willing to run some tests and treat the imbalance. Many endocrinologists do not test T3 and RT3. You may need to consult a holistic MD or an integrative physician that specialize in the subject.

Antithyroid Peroxidase Antibodies

Antithyroid Peroxidase Antibodies or Thyroid Peroxidase antibodies work against thyroid peroxidase which is an enzyme that plays a role in converting T4 to T3. These antibodies can be indicative of tissue destruction that ultimately leads to thyroiditis and Hashimoto's disease. 95% of Hashimoto's disease patients have detectable TPO antibodies. The concentration of TPO antibodies is lower for people with Grave's disease.

- *Thyroglobulin Antibodies*

Testing for these antibodies is relatively common. High levels of thyroglobulin are usually seen in patients with Grave's and Hashimoto's disease. It can also mean that a person is more at risk of developing hypothyroid.

Thyroid-Stimulating Immunoglobulins (TSI) / TSH Stimulating Antibodies (TSAb)

TSI is detected in 90% of Grave's disease patients. The higher the levels of TSI, the more serious the disease is perceived to be. However, the absence of the antibodies does not rule out Grave's disease. Some patients with Hashimoto's disease can also have the antibodies that can lead them to experience hypothyroidism symptoms.

The monitoring of TSI becomes crucial during pregnancy because this can increase the risk of fetal thyroid dysfunction. The antibodies can pass from mother to child through the placenta. Studies shows 10% of pregnant women have elevated TSI antibodies.

Chapter 14:
Problems with Treatments

Doctors usually say that thyroid problems are not easy to diagnose and treat because it can present symptoms that are common to other diseases. A patient may be suffering from unexpected weight gain or fatigue but it can be also misdiagnosed as another disease. Once the doctor suspects that there is some problem with the thyroid, they will usually conduct a TSH test. The problem arises when the diagnosis is solely based on the test results alone. It is still better to take into consideration the clinical examination, symptom reviews as well as thyroid and blood tests before concluding on a diagnosis.

Challenges with Thyroid Diagnosis

Here are some of the challenges that a patient may encounter in having a proper diagnosis:

- *Uninformed doctors*

Unfortunately, patients can no longer solely rely on the knowledge of doctors although their expertise is still valued in diagnosing and treating thyroid problems.

As a patient, be wary of doctors who diagnose a disorder simply by looking at or touching the neck. Feeling for lumps in the neck is only one part of the physical examination that should be conducted by physicians.

They should also perform a thorough clinical thyroid exam and may even check for blood pressure fluctuations and evaluate thyroid symptoms. It is also helpful if the doctor inquires about your medical and family history before diagnosing the disease.

- *Problems in getting tested*

You may find that some doctors are not even willing to run your thyroid tests. Some doctors might think that you are going to use the thyroid results to get thyroid drugs to make you lose weight. Other times, doctors are simply uninformed about the test.

There are patients with thyroid symptoms who get diagnosed with depression and can be prescribed with antidepressants. Some women with hypothyroidism who experience dramatic weight loss and anxiety can be diagnosed as bulimic or anorexic.

Be sure that you are persistent but unemotional when discussing your symptoms with your doctors. Also, it is better if you use descriptions instead of general terms. Instead of saying that you are gaining weight, say that you are gaining weight despite a low calorie diet and regular exercise. You can also say that you experience fatigue despite having 10 hours of sleep each night.

If you are faced with a doctor that refuses to listen to you, then the best option is to look for another one. It might seem ridiculous that you have to struggle just to get lab tests but remember that it is your health that it at risk so keep on insisting. If you are still unable to get a doctor to conduct the tests then you can contact a patient directed laboratory testing service. These laboratory centers allow you to select the blood test that you want and pay them accordingly. The results will be sent directly to you.

- *Your thyroid is normal*

Sometimes, patients will be told that their thyroid tests are normal and that they do not have thyroid problems. There is already a disagreement between doctors about the 'normal' thyroid hormone range so solely relying in TSH test results is not very accurate. Some doctors will suggest to 'wait and see' if the TSH goes up before performing treatment. You can ask about a trial coarse treatment especially if the symptoms are really making you uncomfortable.

- *Fear of Osteoporosis*

Some doctors might fear that treating mild hypothyroidism can increase the risk of osteoporosis. This fear is based on studies that show that long periods of hyperthyroidism treatments is a risk factor of osteoporosis. This reason might lead doctors to delay treatment for hyperthyroidism to avoid that risk.

- *Reliability of the TSH test*

The quality of the TSH test can also be questioned. TSH blood samples are left to sit for several hours before they are sent to laboratories for testing. This can lead to the degradation of the samples. The time of day where blood is extracted can also affect the results. High level of TSH usually occurs in the morning. TSH levels begin to drop throughout the day. This is the reason why some patients may have high hypothyroid levels in the morning but may have normal results later in the day.

A proper diagnosis means that you have to be careful where you have your blood work done. You are also free to ask about the reliability of the test results yourself.

- *Relying too much on TSH results*

Normal TSH levels do not necessarily reflect the total amount of circulating thyroid hormone in the body. You will need complete thyroid blood work that includes Free T3 and Free T4 tests. There are practitioners who feel that thyroid treatment is optimized if the T3 level is on the upper end of the normal range in order to feel well. This means that you also have to get treatment even if you have normal TSH levels but your T3 and T4 is below the normal range.

- *Failure to test for antibodies*

Although autoimmune problems are the most common cause of thyroid problems, some physicians still do not request for antibody test to check for autoimmune disease.

This can be problematic since high levels of thyroid antibodies even if you have normal levels of TSH indicate an autoimmune thyroid disease. The dysfunction might not still be grave to generate symptoms but it can lead to more serious thyroid problems later on.

There are studies that show that treating patients with autoimmune disorder even if they have normal TSH levels can help reduce the severity of the disease progression. Researches also show that it can even stop the development of hypothyroidism.

Is your thyroid medication not working?

After being prescribed with thyroid medicine, you might not notice any improvement in your symptoms. Before you make assumptions that your medicine is not working, you have to explore several factors first.

Make sure that you are taking the right amount of prescribed medicine. Your doctor would probably use the TSH test to determine your response to the medication. It can also take some time before your body adjusts to the medication.

Some patients need to supplement their medication with T3. You might also consider switching brands. However, make sure that you discus your options with your doctors first. You might also feel more comfortable with holistic approach and natural medication.

Lastly, if you do not respond to thyroid treatments despite proper dosage, you may have an adrenal problem. Remember that unless the adrenal problem is dealt with, the thyroid medication will not take effect.

Chapter 15:
About Your Drugs

If your disease has been diagnosed too late or there are no other option but to surgically remove your thyroid or use radioactive iodine, you will need to take thyroid replacement drug to facilitate your hormonal function. Thyroid replacement drug includes synthetic hormones and levothyroxine.

Thyroid Replacement Drugs

- *Levothyroxine*

This is the most prescribed thyroid replacement drug. It is a synthetic form of thyroxine. It is widely available in drug stores and usually come in tablet form. Most doctors recommend branded levothyroxine.

- *Liothyronine*

Thyroid medication manufacturers often make thyroxine and T3 replacement drugs. Liothyronine is a synthetic form of T3. More doctors are prescribing T3 medications. Studies also show that most patients respond better to treatment if additional T3 is added to the medicine.

- *T4/T3 Combination*

There are thyroid drugs that already combine T3 and T4. The most popular is Liotrix which is known in its manufactured form under the brand name Thyrolar.

- *Desiccated Natural Thyroid*

Desiccated thyroid is dried porcine thyroid. Desiccated thyroid is the only drug used during the 1900s before levothyroxine was used. The use of natural thyroid declined in favor of synthetic and modern medicine. However, during and before the 19th century, desiccated thyroid was widely used primarily by older doctors and holistic practitioners who believe that it has better effect than modern drugs. Today, there are still several desiccated thyroid brands available through prescription.

How to take your thyroid medication

Whatever drug you are prescribed with, it is very important that you know how to take it properly.

Doctors always warn their patients not to skip taking their medicine. This is especially true if your thyroid is no longer working and you rely solely on replacement drugs. Even if you only skip one day of medication, it can drastically affect your treatment. Here are some tips in remembering to take your medicine.

- Always make sure that you get what you are prescribed. Do not allow brand or generic substitutions.

- Be consistent on your fiber intake. If you increase or decrease your normal fiber absorption, make sure to get your thyroid rechecked because it can change your body's ability to absorb nutrients.

- Consider placing reminder on your computer or smart phone at the same time of the day to remind you to take your medicine.

- Place your pill container in your desk or any place where you can see it often. However, be sure to keep the drugs away from children and pets.

- Use sticky notes reminders.

- Take the medicine on a particular time of the day so that it can easily become a habit.

- Use a dosette or pill sorter. It is a drug compartment that is usually divided into sections for different days or times of day.

FAQ About How to Take Medicine

Here are some of the frequently asked questions about how to take thyroid medications:

- *Should you take thyroid hormones on an empty stomach?*

Food can delay the absorption of thyroid hormone. Food can also affect the absorption of the drug because it binds within and altering the rate where it dissolves.

Most doctors recommend taking it on an empty stomach and waiting for at least an hour before you eat something.

However, if your lifestyle prevents you from taking it this way, make sure that you are still consistent about taking the medication. If you change the way you take the drugs, you should have another TSH test to see if you are getting the right amount of thyroid hormone. Refrain from constantly changing the way you take your medicine since this can affect the absorption and make it harder for your TSH to regulate properly.

- *What is the impact of high fiber diet?*

Many patients that suffer from thyroid problems may also want to lose weight. Anything that can affect your digestion can affect the absorption of the thyroid hormone in your body. This also includes high fiber diet which can inhibit the absorption of the medication. However, this does not mean that you should stop eating high fiber foods. There are many health benefits associated with fiber. The key is to keep your fiber intake consistent. If you are already consuming a lot of fiber then keep it that way. You can also have a TSH testing done to see if the recommended dosage prescribed to you is appropriate. Do not suddenly increase or decrease your fiber intake while taking thyroid medication or else the amount of hormone absorbed in your body will vary.

- *What is it about iodine and kelp supplements?*

There are many holistic doctors and herbalists that may recommend iodine or kelp supplements for thyroid problems but be very careful in taking it in addition to your thyroid replacement therapy.

The reasoning behind iodine and kelp supplements is that iodine deficiency can cause thyroid disease. Today, iodine deficiency is not very common because most food include iodized salt. In fact, most common forms of thyroid problems are not related to iodine deficiency at all. The thyroids are also very sensitive to iodine and too much can aggravate the thyroid. Some doctors ban their patients from taking iodine supplements in the first place.

- *How about Goitrogenic foods?*

Goitrogenic foods like cauliflower, cauliflower sprouts and turnips acts like antithyroid drugs which can inhibit thyroid function. These types of foods should not be consumed in high amounts by patients who are on thyroid hormone replacement. The enzymes in goitrogenic foods can be destroyed by cooking.

- *Are antacids dangerous?*

Anatacids in liquid or tablet form can reduce the absorption of thyroid drugs. You should not take it with your thyroid hormone. Wait for at least two hours before your take the antacids.

- *Is calcium and calcium fortified juice safe?*

Calcium can also affect the absorption of thyroid drugs. Just like antacids, take it 2-3 hours after your thyroid hormones. This guideline also applies to calcium fortified juices.

- *Should I take over the counter medicine?*

Most labels of over the counter cold, cough and decongestant medicines says that you should not take the medicine if you have thyroid disease. Make sure that you read the package of any medicine that you consume. These drugs contain stimulants which can further aggravate the thyroid. Some people with hypothyroidism are also sensitive to ingredients commonly found in decongestants. Your doctor might only recommend a small dosage to see if it has adverse effect on you and gradually increase the dosage accordingly.

- *Does iron interfere with absorption?*

Iron can interfere with thyroid hormone absorption. This is true whether it is taken alone or is included in your multivitamin. Do not take iron supplements with thyroid hormone and there should be at least two hours in between taking them.

- *What about thyroid hormone and estrogen?*

Women who take estrogen in the form of birth control or hormone replacement may need to increase their thyroid replacement hormone dosage. Estrogen increases the blood proteins in the body which binds to the thyroid hormone and can render it inactive.

Women who have their thyroids surgically removed may need a higher dosage of thyroid replacement hormone. Make sure that you have a TSH test to see if the estrogen has any effect on the thyroid replacement hormone.

What are the important things to know about prescription drugs?

- *Antidepressants*

The use of antidepressants and thyroid hormones at the same time can intensify the effect of both drugs. Make sure

73

that your doctor knows about your antidepressant medication so that he can adjust your dosage.

- *Insulin*

Insulin and other oral hypoglycemic drugs for diabetics can affect thyroid hormones and reduce its effectiveness. Make sure that you watch the period where you start to take thyroid replacement hormone and notice if there is any difference.

- *Cholesterol Lowering Drugs*

Cholesterol lowering drugs bind to the thyroid hormones. Make sure that you take cholesterol lowering hormones 5 hours before or after the thyroid hormones.

- *Anticoagulants*

Anticoagulants become stronger and more potent if thyroid hormone is added. Your doctor may add a new prescription to your thyroid hormone.

Chapter 16:
Troubleshooting Your Thyroid Treatment

There are a lot of factors that can affect your treatment including overmedication, under treatment, heat problems and problems with generic drugs.

Are you overmedicated?

Thyroid replacement hormones usually have few side effects. The most common risk is associated with overmedication. Your tests results can show whether you are taking too much medicine or not. TSH levels that are below normal or at the lower end of the normal range can indicate overmedication. Some doctors can also measure your T4 and T3 levels. If your test results show that you are on the higher side of the normal range, it might mean that you are overmedicated. Elevated pulse rate can also indicate that you might be sensitive to the thyroid hormone.

Symptoms of overmedication

The symptoms of overmedication can vary with each person but it is often similar to the symptoms of hypothyroidism. This includes hair loss, quick pulse, fatigue, irritation, sensitive neck, anxiety and diarrhea.

It can be difficult to recognize the signs of overmedication. Some patients assume that their medicine can make them feel energetic or use it to lose weight but once they start to feel exhausted than normal they may not suspect being overmedicated.

How can a patient be overmedicated?

Here are some ways that you can be overmedicated:

- The dosage prescribed to you is too high. Sometimes, doctors can overestimate the dosage to resolve the symptoms.

- You get an incorrect batch of medicine. You have to pay attention to the symptoms that develop after you get a new refill. The pharmacist may have given you the wrong dosage. Remember that even a slight change in potency of your medicine can have diverse effect.

- You are taking over the counter supplements like animal thyroid. Read the label and see if it includes 'thyroid granular' or adrenal granular'. These supplements can increase the thyroid hormones in your body.

- You lost weight but have not adjusted your thyroid dosage.

- If you just gave birth, your amount of needed thyroid hormones decreases and the same amount of thyroid hormones can be too high during your post-partum period.

- Women who just gave birth may experience fluctuations in thyroid functions and can cause temporary hyperthyroidism.

Dealing with overmedication

The most common solution to overmedication is to reduce the dosage until the blood levels return to normal. You can also be retested and re-evaluate the symptoms until overmedication is resolved.

Under treatment

Patients may still experience thyroid problem symptoms even if their TSH is normal. One cause of this is under treatment. There are two ways under treatment can happen. First, some doctors only prescribe low dosage just to get the patient to a normal TSH level. Second, your current thyroid treatment is not enough and you might need T3 supplements in order to feel well.

How to cope with under treatment

If you still feel the symptoms of hypothyroidism despite regular treatment, the first thing that you can do is to document the symptoms that you are feeling. This will make it easier for your doctor to evaluate your condition. If the doctor refuses to discuss or consider other forms of therapy without providing a substantial reason, then you may need to look for another doctor.

Should you be concerned about taking generic medication?

Most doctors advise against the use of generic thyroid medication. Patients usually consider the cost difference and use generic medicine. However, while some people think that generic medicine is equivalent to branded preparations; it is still not proven that they have the same therapeutic benefit.

Levothyroxine, a drug commonly used to treat thyroid problems, vary in terms of potency depending on the manufacturer. This is the reason why it is best if you stick with the same brand to avoid potency variation.

Generic levothyroxine can also be consistent in potency but your doctor is unable to prescribe the specific product that you will get. Basically, the patient can get the same medicine from different manufacturers with each prescription refill and can lead to potency fluctuations.

What should you do?

You have to be very consistent in taking your medication. You should always check your prescriptions each time you get it. Do not assume that you have the same prescription without confirming it.

Hot temperature can be hazardous to your medicine

Extreme temperature can also affect your prescription drugs. Storing your medicine at high temperature can degrade its quality and stability. The recommended temperature for most medicine is 77 degrees F. Summer heat can expose the medicine and degrade your drugs even without you being aware of it.

Thyroid medicine manufacturers advise their clients to replace their medication if it has been exposed 86 degrees for a length of time.

How to protect your medication?

You can protect your medicines with these tips in mind:

- Check the storage information in the label of the medicine to ensure that you are storing it properly.

- Place your medicine in your hand carry luggage when you travel on a plane instead of placing it in a checked luggage. Make sure that your prescriptions drugs are labeled to assist with the screening process.

- If you are traveling in a car, do not place your medicine in the trunk and do not leave it for a long period of time.

- Make sure that the pharmacies where you purchase your medicine do not turn off the air conditioning when it closes.

Chapter 17:
Living with Thyroid Problems

Managing the symptoms of thyroid problems may require time, patience and sacrifice. Living with thyroid problems can easily depress patients most especially if their thyroid gland is destroyed or removed.

Ways to stay energized

Even patients who get proper treatment can experience fatigue. Here are some tips in staying energized.

- *Take your medication*

Most patients respond well to hypothyroid medication. This is especially true if the medicine is taken as prescribed by the doctor. Even severe cases of hypothyroidism can improve within six months if the treatment is right. T3 and T4 medication can also be recommended for people who still continue to experience fatigue even with regular treatment.

- *Balance your diet*

Most holistic doctors say that a well balanced diet can do more good for the body than medicine. It is true that eating a diet rich in whole foods can drastically increase the recovery rate for most patients. Whole foods contain vitamins and minerals that can strengthen the body and promote body function.

- *Try cognitive behavioral therapy*

Cognitive therapy is a psychological therapy that aims to change negative habits and replace it with more positive thoughts. Studies show that this therapy can help people be more physically active and combat anxiety and fatigue. Cognitive therapy can help change your mindset and prevent negativity.

- *Limit alcohol and caffeine*

If you are having problems with hypothyroidism, it is easy to use caffeine and alcohol to control your energy levels. However, caffeine can only energize you for a short time and it does not address long term fatigue problems. Caffeine and alcohol also prevents the normal sleep cycle.

- *Engage in physical activity*

Some patients with thyroid problems think that they do not have enough energy for exercise but it can actually counter fatigue and increase energy levels during the day and improve sleep quality at night. You can start by exercising for 30 minutes in a day then gradually increase the intensity as you get better.

- *Take extra steps to ensure that you sleep better*

Getting enough sleep is essential to everyone. Good quality sleeps can fight fatigue caused by hypothyroidism. Make sure that your bedroom is conducive for sleeping.

- *Avoid Nicotine*

Nicotine is a stimulant which can interfere with your sleeping pattern. It is also known to interfere with your thyroid treatment. Patients who quit smoking found that after they get pass the withdrawal symptom they are able to sleep better.

Decrease Joint Pain Caused by Hypothyroidism

Joint pain is a common complaint among people with hypothyroidism. There are certain aspects and therapies that can help you ease the pain. Hypothyroidism slows down the metabolism and can affect your muscles as well. People with severe hypothyroidism are susceptible to joint swelling and pain.

- *Try low impact aerobics*

20-60 minutes of daily aerobic exercise can increase your heart rate and speed up your metabolism. This can help you lose weight and reduce the risk of joint pain. Try the elliptical machine instead of the treadmill for a low impact exercise. Swimming is also beneficial for people with weak joints.

- *Strengthen your muscles*

Strength exercises that can build muscle are beneficial for people with hypothyroidism. Muscles burn more calories even at rest and can also relive strain in your joints. Stronger muscles also support the knees. Start slow then gradually add more repetitions as you become stronger.

- *Omega 3 fatty acid*

Foods rich in Omega 3 fatty acid can reduce inflammation in your joints. Most coldwater fish like salmon, tuna and mackerel are rich source of Omega 3 fatty acids.

How to deal with the emotions of Hypothyroidism

Being diagnosed with hypothyroidism can have two effects on a person. On one hand, the patient might feel relieved because their symptoms of depression, lethargy, weight gain and aches are formally categorized as symptoms of a disorder and it is not only in their head. However, hypothyroidism medication can be slow acting so it may take some time before a person starts to feel better physically and emotionally.

You do not need to sit around and wait until your medication takes effect. You can also deal with anxiety and other emotions related to hypothyroidism.

- *Talk to your therapists*

Talking to a therapist can help if you are concerned about your emotions and experience difficulty in sleeping or eating. Therapists can help you work through your emotional issues and how to resolve them.

- *Reduce stress*

Stress can aggravate any medical condition. You will also respond better to treatment if you are not stressed out. Always make time to relax and unwind. It can be as simple as having dinner with your friends or watching a funny movie. Also, another great way to manage stress is to avoid taking more that you are capable. Set comfortable limits when it comes to your work and personal life.

- *Get a massage*

Massages can be seen as a luxury but it is very effective in reducing stress. It can loosen tight muscles and lift your mood instantly. It is also a great way to have some peace and quiet.

- *Be social*

Enjoying time with your family and friends is a sure way to improve your mood. This can help combat lethargy and depression.

How to get support for thyroid problems

Everyone who is diagnosed with a disease can suffer from negative emotional effects. It can take some time before the effect of drugs can take place so someone with thyroid problems needs the support of their family and friends to live well. Here are the people who should be part of your support team:

- *The doctor*

Your doctor is your partner in managing your thyroid problem. They are the ones who are responsible for dispensing medication and monitoring your condition. Your doctors should know how the disease is affecting you and can explain the symptoms properly.

- *Your family*

It is also important to inform your family about your condition. Since thyroid problem can be passed from one generation to another, your family members may want to be tested too. Also, telling your family about your condition can help them understand what you are going through. Tell them about your symptoms such as depression, fatigue or anxiety. More importantly, you family's encouragement is a great source of support for you.

- *Your therapists*

If you decide to consult your therapist about your depression or emotional problems, do not forget to keep them informed about your medical standing as well. This will give them a good idea about how your disease is affecting your mental and emotional health. A psychiatrist can also prescribe medicines that are compatible with your thyroid medication.

- *A support groups*

Support groups are becoming more popular as a source of motivation and encouragement for people with different problems. Joining a support group that consists of people with the same medical condition can help you express yourself and find people who understand what you are going through. You can even share great ideas and tips.

- *Enlist the help of an exercise buddy*

Exercise is an important part of managing thyroid problems. Enlist the help of an exercise buddy to motivate you to work out. You are more likely to show up if you know that someone is waiting for you.

How to look your best with thyroid problems

Thyroid problem can affect how you look physically and can make you look unhealthy. Fortunately, there are some things that you can do to prevent thyroid problems from cramping your personal style.

Coping with extreme dry skin

Lack of hormones can make your skin look and feel dry. Here are some of the things that you can do:

- Moisturize. Moisturizing your skin using creams and lotions can ease dryness. Choose products that work well with your skin. Organic skin products tend to have the best benefit because they do not contain harmful ingredients that can seep into your skin. Skin moisturizer is best applied after you have cleansed your skin.

- Hydrate. Drinking water can hydrate your skin from the inside. It also helps flush toxins out of your body.

- Turn down the heat. You can bath in cool water instead of hot water. Hot water tends to dry the skin quickly. Also, it is best if your pat your skin dry rather than rubbing it.

Coping with thinning hair

Hair loss due to thyroid problems is usually mild. Be sure that your loss of hair is because of your thyroid problem and not other factors like stress, iron loss and aging. Hair loss that is caused by other factors besides thyroid problems cannot be solved by thyroid therapy. For thyroid problems related to thyroid, you can try these solutions:

- Hair and scalp treatment. There are many over the counter treatment that can help strengthen your hair.

- Be gentle. Do not tug or pull your hair often. You should also avoid exposing it to many chemicals.

- Consider cover ups. You can be stylish and use hats, wigs or scarves as cover-ups.

Coping with eye puffiness

Eye puffiness is one effect of hypothyroidism. Make sure that you drink a lot of water. You can also use a cold pack to relive the swelling in your eyes.

Chapter 18:
What Can You Do To Promote Awareness

People who have been through a lot because of their thyroid problems may want to help spread thyroid awareness. Some people feel that it is part of their responsibility to help other people if they can. Here are some of the things that you can do to promote awareness:

Share information with friends and relatives

If you find a friend or a relative that is struggling with symptoms of thyroid problem like weight gain, depression or fatigue, make sure that you mention thyroid disease. You can relay the information that you know and send some links and resources to them.

Get thyroid newsletters and spread the word

It is fortunate that more and more people are becoming aware of thyroid problems. There are medical sites that specialize in thyroid problems and provide health articles for patients. Signing up for newsletters can keep you updated about the latest medical research.

Promote books on thyroid disease

Books in your local libraries can help people who want to learn more about the disease. You can also encourage your local library to keep a stock of books related to thyroid disease. You can even donate the books yourself. This generous act can help the lives of other people in your area.

Provide support

Providing support for other thyroid patients is a crucial factor in spreading awareness. You can show your support by attending group support meetings or spreading the word on your social media accounts.

You can also provide personal support for thyroid disease patients. Some hospitals allow support groups to visit patients. You can also start your own group if there are still none in your local area. Consider donating time or money to non-profit groups that advocate thyroid awareness. Your moral support can greatly help other people who go through difficult times.

Conclusion

Thank you again for buying

"Thyroid Health: Ultimate Guide that will cure your thyroid problems"

I hope this book was able to help you to understand the process of investigating your options in relation to cure your thyroid symptoms.

The next procedure is to take some time to consider your options carefully and think about the next steps, one important fact to reiterate at this stage is that this book has provided you with some generic information on the subject, it was never intended to and certainly does not replace medical advice from a professional, before making any lifestyle changes please ensure you consult your physician.

All what's left to say is Good Luck, with a positive attitude and determination you can reach your goals and get that life you've always wanted.

Once again,

Thank you and good luck!

Lucas Ether

www.ingramcontent.com/pod-product-compliance
Lightning Source LLC
Chambersburg PA
CBHW050419290526
45786CB00003B/1323